HEALTHY AND POISON FOOD COMBO

Health wellness

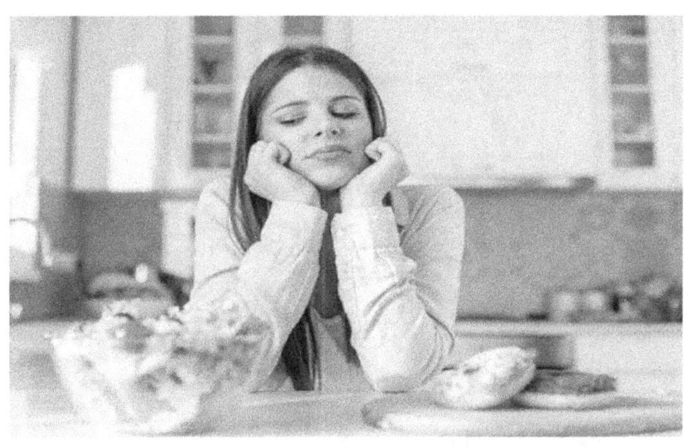

Introduction

Once upon a time, in a quaint town nestled between rolling hills, lived a man named Oliver. Known for his adventurous palate, Oliver took pride in experimenting with unique food combinations. One fateful day, he decided to create a dish that blended flavors in ways that had never been attempted before.

In his small kitchen, Oliver gathered an assortment of ingredients: spicy peppers, sweet fruits, rich cheeses, and exotic spices. With unwavering confidence, he concocted a dish that seemed like a masterpiece on his taste buds. Ignoring traditional culinary wisdom, he devoured the unconventional fusion.

As the hours passed, Oliver began to feel an unsettling discomfort in his stomach. The once vibrant hues of the dish now seemed like a harbinger of his impending doom. Ignoring the warning signs, he dismissed the discomfort as mere indigestion.

However, the combination of incompatible ingredients took a toll on his digestive system. Agony gripped him, and his condition worsened rapidly. Panicking, Oliver sought medical attention, but it was too late. The doctors struggled to understand the unusual mix of elements wreaking havoc inside him.

With regret and sorrow, Oliver succumbed to the consequences of his daring culinary experiment. The town mourned the loss of their adventurous food enthusiast, a cautionary tale echoing through the streets about the importance of respecting the delicate balance of flavors in the pursuit of gastronomic pleasure.

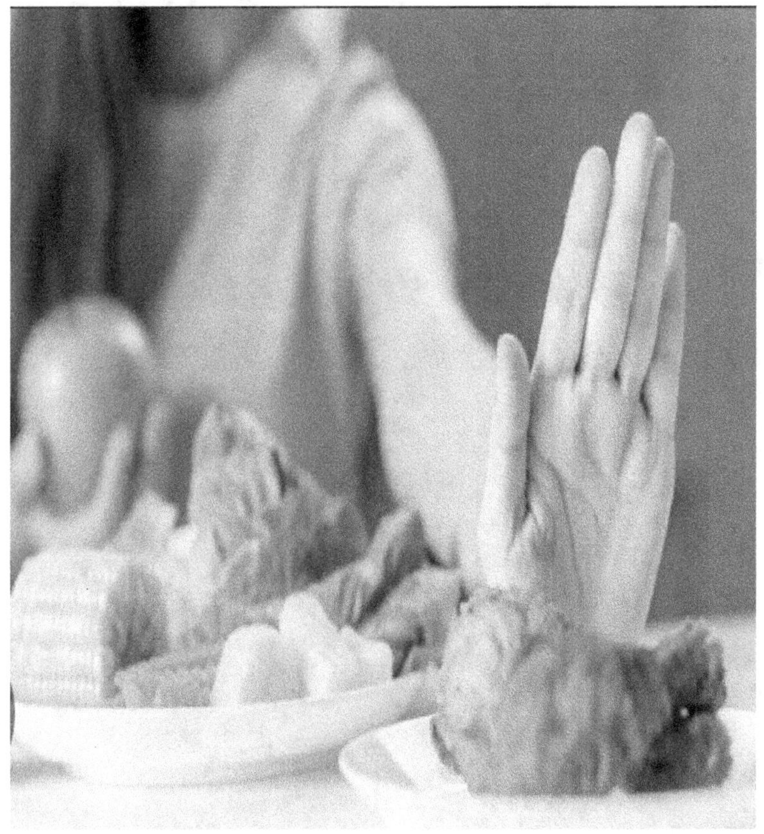

Table of Contents:

Introduction

CHAPTER 1: Purpose of Food Combinations

Impact on Digestion

CHAPTER 2 : Basic Principles of Food Combinations

Understanding Macronutrients

Balancing Proteins, Carbohydrates, and Fats

CHAPTER 3: Optimal Pairings

Protein and Vegetables: A Nutrient-Rich Duo

Carbohydrates and Fiber: Essential Components for a Healthy Diet

Fats and Essential Nutrients

CHAPTER 4 : Incompatible Combinations

Avoiding Conflicting Food Groups

Common Mistakes in Food Combining

CHAPTER 5: Enhancing Nutrient Absorption

Synergistic Food Pairings

Bioavailability and Nutrient Utilization: Unveiling the Intricacies of Nutrient Absorption

CHAPTER 1: Purpose of Food Combinations

Food combinations play a crucial role in optimizing nutrient absorption, digestion, and overall well-being. The purpose of carefully pairing foods goes beyond taste preferences; it extends to promoting optimal health and energy. Here are key aspects of the purpose of food combinations:

1. Enhanced Nutrient Absorption:

   - Combining certain foods can enhance the absorption of nutrients. For example, consuming vitamin C-rich foods with iron-rich ones improves the absorption of iron.

- Including healthy fats with vegetables can aid in the absorption of fat-soluble vitamins like A, D, E, and K.

2. Balanced Macronutrients:

- Combining carbohydrates, proteins, and fats in a balanced way helps maintain stable blood sugar levels, providing sustained energy and preventing energy crashes.

- Pairing complex carbohydrates with lean proteins or healthy fats can contribute to a more balanced and sustained release of energy.

3. Improved Digestion:

- Some foods digest at different rates, and combining them strategically can optimize the overall digestion process.

- Pairing easily digestible foods with slower-digesting ones can help regulate the release of nutrients and prevent digestive discomfort.

4. Blood Sugar Regulation:

- Combining fiber-rich carbohydrates with proteins and fats can slow down the absorption of glucose, helping to stabilize blood sugar levels.

- This is particularly important for individuals with diabetes or those aiming to manage their weight effectively.

5. Synergistic Antioxidant Effects:

- Combining foods with diverse antioxidants can create a synergistic effect, enhancing the overall antioxidant capacity of the diet.

- For example, pairing tomatoes with olive oil boosts the absorption of lycopene, a powerful antioxidant in tomatoes.

6. Gut Health Optimization:

- Certain food combinations support a healthy gut microbiome. Including prebiotics (found in foods like garlic, onions, and bananas) with probiotics (found in fermented foods) promotes a thriving gut environment.

7. Reduced Digestive Stress:

- Avoiding incompatible food combinations, such as combining high-starch foods with acidic fruits, can prevent digestive discomfort and bloating.

- Proper food combining may alleviate common digestive issues like indigestion and gas.

8. Optimal Weight Management:

- Thoughtful food combinations can contribute to weight management by promoting satiety and preventing overeating.

- Combining lean proteins, high-fiber foods, and healthy fats can create satisfying meals that support weight loss or maintenance.

In summary, the purpose of food combinations extends beyond taste and cultural preferences. By understanding how different foods interact in the body, individuals can make informed choices to enhance nutrient absorption, support digestion, regulate blood sugar, and promote overall health and well-being.

Impact on Digestion

Digestion plays a crucial role in the overall health of an individual, influencing various aspects of the body. The impact on digestion is multifaceted, influenced by dietary choices, lifestyle factors, and underlying health conditions. Understanding these factors can contribute to maintaining a healthy digestive system.

1. Dietary Habits:

- **Nutrient Intake**: Consuming a balanced diet rich in fiber, vitamins, and minerals supports optimal digestion. Fiber aids in regular bowel movements and prevents constipation.

- **Hydration**: An adequate intake of water is essential for digestion. Water helps in the breakdown of food, absorption of nutrients, and smooth movement of stools through the digestive tract.

- **Processed Foods**: High intake of processed and refined foods can contribute to digestive issues. These foods often lack essential nutrients and fiber, leading to irregular bowel habits.

2. **Lifestyle Factors**:

- **Physical Activity**: Regular exercise promotes healthy digestion by enhancing bowel movements and reducing the risk of conditions like constipation.

- **Meal Timing**: Irregular eating patterns or consuming large meals can affect digestion negatively. Maintaining consistent meal times supports a more regulated digestive process.

- **Stress Management**: Stress can impact digestion through the gut-brain connection. Chronic stress may lead to conditions such as irritable bowel syndrome (IBS) or exacerbate existing digestive issues.

3. Gut Microbiota:

- **Microbial Balance**: The gut microbiota, composed of trillions of microorganisms, plays a pivotal role in digestion. An imbalance in these microbes can lead to conditions like dysbiosis, affecting nutrient absorption and immune function.

- **Probiotics**: Introducing beneficial bacteria through probiotics can positively influence digestion. Probiotic-rich foods and supplements contribute to a healthy gut microbiome.

4. Digestive Disorders:

   - **Inflammatory Bowel Disease (IBD):** Conditions like Crohn's disease and ulcerative colitis can severely impact digestion, leading to inflammation, abdominal pain, and altered bowel habits.

   - **Gastroesophageal Reflux Disease (GERD)**: GERD can cause acid reflux, affecting the esophagus and leading to discomfort and potential damage to the digestive tract.

5. Aging and Digestion:

   - **Slower Digestive Process**: Aging can slow down digestion, affecting nutrient absorption and bowel regularity. Adequate nutrition and hydration become crucial in maintaining digestive health for older individuals.

6. Medications:

- Antibiotics and Digestive Health: Certain medications, especially antibiotics, can disrupt the balance of gut bacteria, potentially leading to digestive issues such as diarrhea.

In conclusion, the impact on digestion is a complex interplay of various factors. Adopting a well-balanced diet, incorporating healthy lifestyle practices, managing stress, and addressing underlying health conditions contribute to maintaining optimal digestive health. Regular check-ups with healthcare professionals can help identify and address any digestive issues promptly.

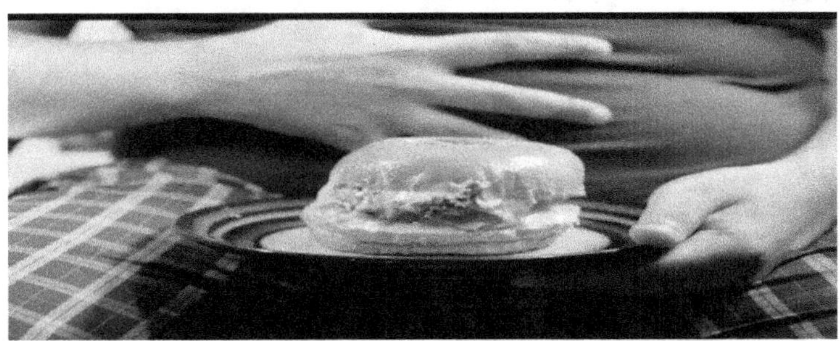

CHAPTER 2 : Basic Principles of Food Combinations

Eating a well-balanced and nutritious diet involves not only selecting the right foods but also understanding how to combine them effectively. The principles of food combinations can significantly impact digestion, nutrient absorption, and overall health. Here are some fundamental guidelines to consider:

1. Balanced Macronutrients:

  - Ensure meals contain a balance of carbohydrates, proteins, and fats.

- This balance helps regulate blood sugar levels, providing sustained energy and promoting satiety.

2. Timing Matters:

- Consume a mix of macronutrients throughout the day rather than heavily favoring one group in a single meal.

- Distribute meals and snacks evenly to maintain a steady energy level.

3. Complementary Proteins:

- Combine different protein sources to ensure a complete range of essential amino acids.

- Examples include combining beans and rice or hummus and whole-grain pita.

4. Favor Whole Foods:

- Choose whole, minimally processed foods over refined and processed options.

- Whole foods often contain a broader spectrum of nutrients and fiber.

5. Synergistic Nutrient Pairing:

- Some nutrients enhance the absorption of others. For instance, pairing vitamin C-rich foods with iron-rich foods can boost iron absorption.

- Combining healthy fats with fat-soluble vitamins enhances their absorption.

6. Mindful Food Combining:

- Pay attention to how certain foods make you feel when combined.

- Some people find that certain combinations aid digestion, while others may cause discomfort.

7. Digestive Enzymes:

- Consider the digestive enzymes present in different foods.

- For instance, fruits are generally easier to digest when consumed separately from protein-rich meals.

8. Food Combining for Digestive Comfort:

- Some follow principles like "food combining for better digestion," which suggests separating certain food groups to promote optimal digestion and reduce bloating.

9. Variety and Colorful Plates:

- Incorporate a variety of colors in your meals to ensure a diverse range of nutrients.

- Different colors often indicate various phytonutrients with unique health benefits.

10. Hydration with Meals:

- Sip water with meals to aid digestion, but avoid excessive consumption, which may dilute digestive enzymes.

11. Individual Tolerance:

- Pay attention to your body's response to different food combinations.

- Individual tolerance can vary, so it's essential to find what works best for you.

By understanding and applying these basic principles of food combinations, you can create meals that not only taste good but also support optimal nutrition and digestive health. Remember that individual needs and preferences may vary, so it's crucial to listen to your body and make adjustments accordingly.

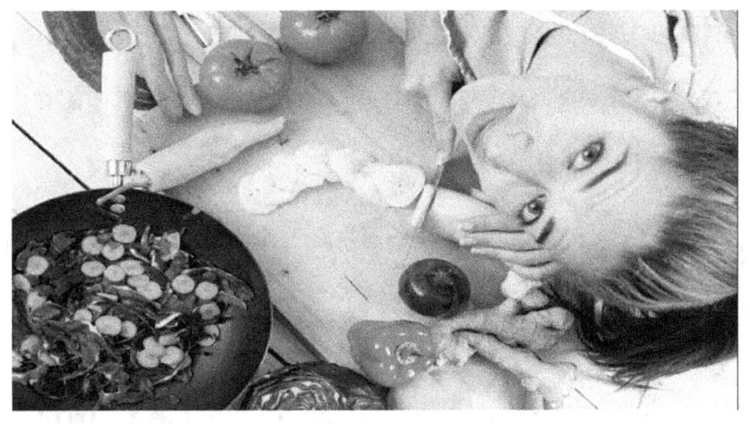

Understanding Macronutrients

Macronutrients are essential components of the human diet that provide the energy and building blocks necessary for optimal bodily functions. Comprising carbohydrates, proteins, and fats, these macronutrients play distinct roles in supporting overall health and well-being.

1. Carbohydrates:

- **Function**: Carbohydrates are the primary source of energy for the body. They are broken down into glucose, which fuels various cellular activities.

- **Types**: There are two main types of carbohydrates: simple carbohydrates (sugars) and complex carbohydrates (starches and fibers). Whole grains, fruits, and vegetables are excellent sources of complex carbs, providing sustained energy.

2. Proteins:

- **Function**: Proteins are crucial for the growth, repair, and maintenance of tissues and organs. They are composed of amino acids, the building blocks of the body.

- **Sources**: Proteins can be derived from both animal and plant sources. Animal products like meat, eggs, and dairy are rich in complete proteins, while plant-based sources include beans, legumes, and nuts.

3. Fats:

- **Function**: Fats play a key role in hormone production, cell structure, and absorption of fat-soluble vitamins (A, D, E, K). They also serve as an energy reserve.

- **Types**: There are saturated fats (found in animal products), unsaturated fats (monounsaturated and polyunsaturated), and trans fats (commonly found in processed foods). A balanced intake of healthy fats, such as those from avocados, olive oil, and fatty fish, is essential.

Understanding the balance and proportions of these macronutrients is vital for maintaining a healthy diet. The optimal distribution of macronutrients can vary based on individual factors like age, gender, activity level, and overall health goals. It's often recommended to follow a balanced diet that includes a variety of nutrient-dense foods.

4. Caloric Value:

- **Calories**: Each macronutrient provides a certain number of calories per gram—carbohydrates and proteins contribute 4 calories per gram, while fats provide 9 calories per gram. Monitoring caloric intake is essential for weight management.

5. Balancing Macronutrients:

- **Individual Needs**: The ideal macronutrient ratio varies among individuals. Athletes may require a higher proportion of carbohydrates for energy, while those aiming for weight loss might focus on a higher protein intake to support muscle maintenance.

6. Dietary Guidelines:

- **Nutrient-Dense Foods**: Emphasizing nutrient-dense foods ensures that the body receives essential vitamins and minerals along with macronutrients. This includes a variety of fruits, vegetables, lean proteins, and whole grains.

7. Health Implications:

- **Imbalances**: Consuming an excess of any macronutrient can lead to health issues. For instance, excessive intake of saturated fats may contribute to cardiovascular problems, while inadequate protein can impair muscle function.

In conclusion, understanding macronutrients is fundamental to making informed dietary choices. Tailoring macronutrient intake to individual needs and goals promotes overall health and well-being. A balanced diet that includes a variety of nutrient-rich foods ensures the body receives the necessary components for optimal functioning.

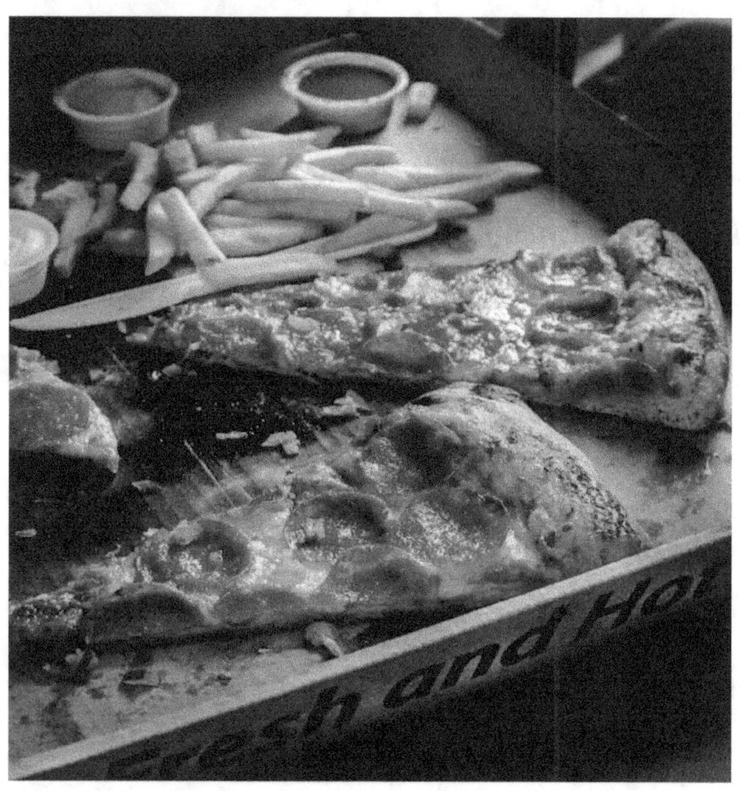

Balancing Proteins, Carbohydrates, and Fats

Balancing proteins, carbohydrates, and fats is essential for maintaining a healthy and well-rounded diet. Each of these macronutrients plays a unique role in the body, and their proper combination is crucial for optimal nutrition.

1. Proteins:

Proteins are the building blocks of the body, involved in the repair and growth of tissues. Including a variety of protein sources such as lean meats, fish, eggs, dairy, legumes, and plant-based proteins ensures a diverse range of essential amino acids. Aim for a daily intake that aligns with your activity level and body weight.

2. Carbohydrates:

Carbohydrates are the body's primary energy source. Opt for complex carbohydrates found in whole grains, fruits, vegetables, and legumes rather than simple sugars. This provides sustained energy, supports digestive health, and helps regulate blood sugar levels. Fiber-rich choices also contribute to feelings of fullness and assist in weight management.

3. Fats:

Healthy fats are crucial for various bodily functions, including hormone production and absorption of fat-soluble vitamins. Incorporate sources of unsaturated fats like avocados, nuts, seeds, and olive oil. Limit saturated and trans fats found in processed foods and certain animal products to promote heart health.

Tips for Balancing:

1. Portion Control: Be mindful of portion sizes to prevent overconsumption of any macronutrient.

2. Meal Timing: Distribute macronutrients throughout the day to maintain energy levels and support metabolism. Aim for balanced meals and snacks.

3. Hydration: Stay adequately hydrated, as water plays a vital role in nutrient absorption and overall well-being.

4. Individual Needs: Consider personal factors such as age, activity level, and health goals when determining the ideal macronutrient ratio.

5. Variety: Embrace a diverse range of foods to ensure a broad spectrum of nutrients. This helps prevent nutrient deficiencies and supports overall health. Balancing proteins, carbohydrates, and fats is not a one-size-fits-all approach. Consulting with a nutrition professional can provide personalized guidance based on individual needs and preferences. Ultimately, a well-balanced diet promotes overall health, energy, and longevity.

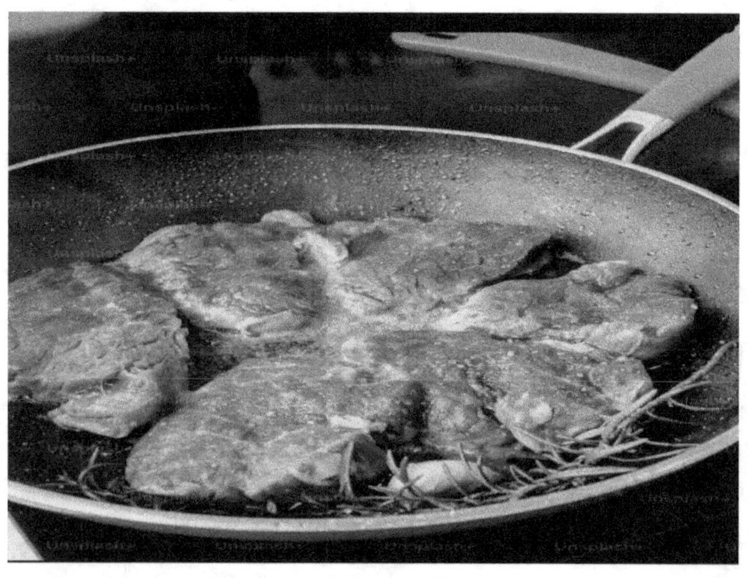

CHAPTER 3: Optimal Pairings

Optimal food pairings involve combining ingredients that complement each other in flavor, texture, and nutritional value. Crafting harmonious combinations can enhance the overall dining experience. Here's a comprehensive guide to optimal food pairings:

1. Flavor Harmony:

   - **Contrast and Balance**: Pairing sweet with savory, or spicy with creamy, creates a balance that stimulates the palate.

   - **Complementary Flavors**: Match ingredients with complimentary tastes, such as pairing acidic tomatoes with rich, umami-packed cheese.

2. Texture Contrast:

- **Crunch and Creaminess**: Combining textures like the crunch of nuts with the creaminess of a sauce adds a delightful contrast.

- **Tender with Crispy**: Pairing tender proteins with crispy coatings provides a satisfying textural interplay.

3. Cultural Affinities:

- **Regional Pairings:** Explore traditional pairings from specific cuisines, like pasta with tomato sauce in Italian cuisine or rice with curry in Asian dishes.

- **Global Fusion**: Experiment with combining elements from different culinary traditions for unique and exciting flavors.

4. Wine and Food Pairing:

- **Reds with Reds, Whites with Whites**: Match the intensity of wines with the richness of the dish. Red wines often pair well with robust meats, while whites complement lighter fare.

5. Seasonal Pairings:

  - **Fresh and Seasonal Ingredients**: Opt for ingredients that are in season together. This ensures the flavors are at their peak and harmonize naturally.

6. Nutritional Synergy:

- **Complete Proteins**: Combine plant-based proteins like beans and rice to create a complete amino acid profile.

  - **Vitamin and Mineral Pairings**: Enhance nutrient absorption by pairing foods rich in certain vitamins with those containing complementary minerals.

7. Temperature Balance:

- **Hot and Cold Contrasts**: Serve warm dishes with cool accompaniments, creating a dynamic experience for the taste buds.

8. Mindful Pairing:

- **Mindful Eating**: Consider the nutritional benefits of each component to create a well-rounded and satisfying meal.

- **Personal Preferences**: Tailor pairings to individual tastes, taking into account dietary restrictions and preferences.

9. Dessert Pairings:

- **Sweet and Salty**: The classic combination of sweet and salty can be explored in desserts, such as caramel with sea salt.

10. Experimental Pairings:

- **Unexpected Combinations**: Don't be afraid to experiment with unconventional pairings, discovering new and exciting flavor profiles.

Remember that these guidelines serve as a foundation, and personal preferences play a significant role in creating optimal food pairings. Whether you're planning a meal for yourself or hosting a dinner party, experimenting with different combinations can lead to delightful culinary discoveries.

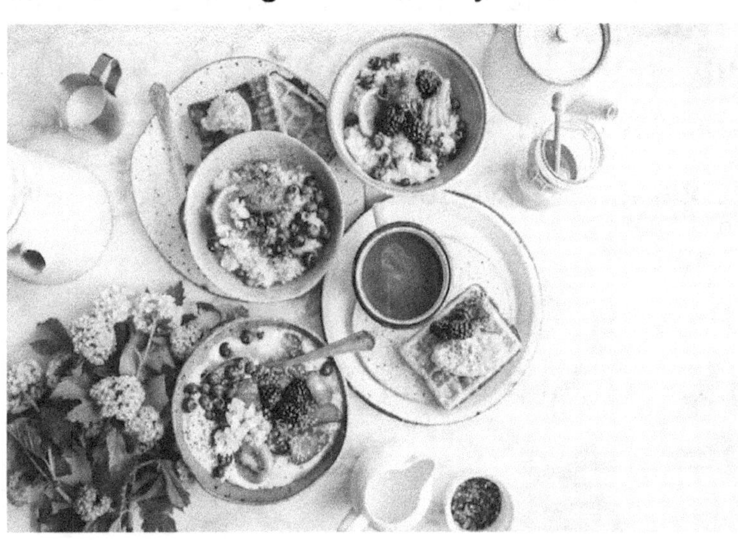

Protein and Vegetables: A Nutrient-Rich Duo

Protein and vegetables form a powerful partnership in promoting overall health and well-being. Both are essential components of a balanced diet, providing a myriad of nutrients that support various bodily functions. Let's delve into the benefits, sources, and importance of incorporating protein and vegetables into your daily meals.

Protein:

1. Essential Building Blocks:

- Proteins are crucial macronutrients composed of amino acids, the building blocks of life.

- These amino acids play a pivotal role in building and repairing tissues, supporting immune function, and producing enzymes and hormones.

2. Dietary Sources:

- Animal sources: Lean meats, poultry, fish, eggs, and dairy products are rich in complete proteins containing all essential amino acids.

- Plant sources: Legumes, beans, nuts, seeds, tofu, and certain grains offer plant-based protein options. Combining different plant sources can help achieve a complete amino acid profile.

3. Muscle Health:

- Protein is especially vital for muscle health, supporting muscle growth, repair, and maintenance.

- Athletes and individuals engaged in regular physical activity often require increased protein intake to meet their body's demands.

4. Satiety and Weight Management:

- Protein-rich foods contribute to a feeling of fullness, aiding in weight management by reducing overall caloric intake.

- Including protein in meals can help regulate appetite and prevent overeating.

Vegetables:

1. Nutrient Powerhouses:

- Vegetables are nutrient-dense, packed with vitamins, minerals, fiber, and antioxidants that support various bodily functions.

- Different colored vegetables provide a diverse array of nutrients, each with unique health benefits.

2. Fiber and Digestive Health:

- Vegetables are an excellent source of dietary fiber, promoting digestive health and preventing constipation.

- Fiber also contributes to a feeling of satiety, aiding in weight management.

3. Disease Prevention:

- Regular consumption of vegetables is associated with a lower risk of chronic diseases, including heart disease, certain cancers, and diabetes.

- Antioxidants in vegetables help neutralize free radicals, protecting cells from damage.

4. Versatility in Cooking:

- Vegetables offer versatility in culinary creations, enhancing flavor, texture, and visual appeal in various dishes.

- Incorporating a variety of vegetables ensures a diverse nutrient intake.

Synergy in the Plate:

1. Balanced Nutrition:

- Combining protein and vegetables in meals creates a balanced nutritional profile, supplying essential nutrients for overall health.

- This combination supports sustained energy levels, muscle health, and overall well-being.

2. Meal Ideas:

- Grilled chicken with a colorful array of roasted vegetables, lentil soup with a side salad, or a tofu stir-fry with mixed vegetables are examples of balanced protein and vegetable meals.

In conclusion, embracing a diet rich in both protein and vegetables is a key strategy for promoting optimal health. Whether your preference leans towards animal or plant-based sources, incorporating a variety of protein and vegetables into your diet ensures a spectrum of nutrients essential for a thriving and resilient body.

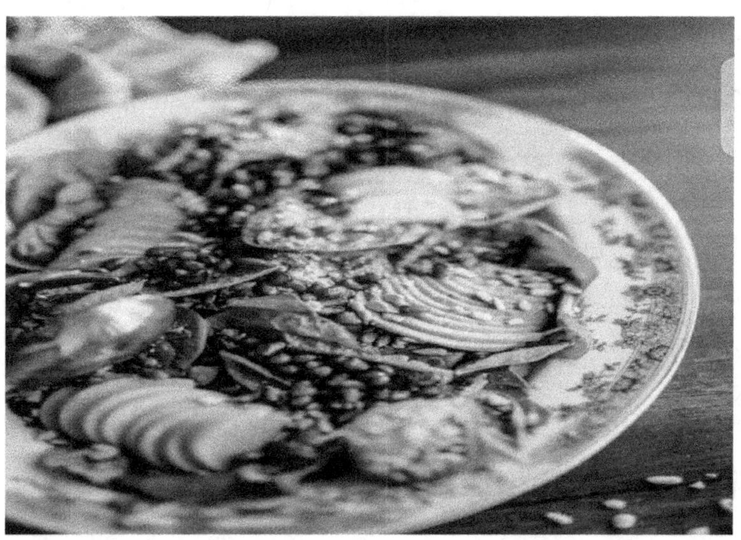

Carbohydrates and Fiber: Essential Components for a Healthy Diet

Carbohydrates are a vital macronutrient found in a variety of foods, playing a crucial role in providing energy for the body. Comprising sugars, starches, and fibers, carbohydrates are classified into simple and complex forms. Simple carbohydrates, like those found in fruits and refined sugars, provide quick energy, while complex carbohydrates, present in whole grains and legumes, release energy more gradually.

Types of Carbohydrates:

1. **Monosaccharides**: Single sugar molecules like glucose and fructose.

2. **Disaccharides**: Pairs of monosaccharides, such as sucrose (glucose + fructose) and lactose (glucose + galactose).

3. **Polysaccharides**: Complex carbohydrates, consisting of long chains of glucose units. Examples include starch (found in grains and vegetables) and glycogen (stored in muscles and the liver).

Importance of Carbohydrates:

1. **Energy Source**: Primary fuel for the body, especially vital for brain function.

2. **Protein Sparing:** Allows proteins to focus on their structural and enzymatic roles instead of being used for energy.

Fiber: The Indigestible Hero:

Fiber is a type of carbohydrate that the body cannot digest or absorb. It comes in two main forms: soluble and insoluble.

1. Soluble Fiber:

- Found in foods like oats, beans, and fruits.

- Forms a gel-like substance in the digestive tract, aiding in cholesterol regulation and blood sugar control.

- Supports a healthy gut microbiota.

2. Insoluble Fiber:

- Present in wheat bran, vegetables, and whole grains.

- Adds bulk to stool, preventing constipation and promoting digestive regularity.

- Offers a feeling of fullness, assisting in weight management.

Health Benefits of Fiber:

1. Digestive Health:** Prevents constipation, diverticulitis, and other digestive issues.

2. **Heart Health**: Soluble fiber helps lower cholesterol levels, reducing the risk of heart disease.

3. **Blood Sugar Control**: Slows the absorption of sugar, beneficial for individuals with diabetes.

4. **Weight Management**: Adds volume to meals, promoting satiety and reducing overall calorie intake.

Balancing Carbohydrates and Fiber in Your Diet:

1. **Whole Foods**: Prioritize whole, unprocessed foods like fruits, vegetables, whole grains, and legumes.

2. **Limit Added Sugars**: Minimize intake of sugary beverages and processed foods.

3. Read Labels: Be aware of food labels to identify sources of both beneficial and harmful carbohydrates.

In conclusion, understanding the role of carbohydrates and incorporating a balance of both simple and complex forms, along with an adequate intake of fiber, is essential for maintaining overall health and well-being.

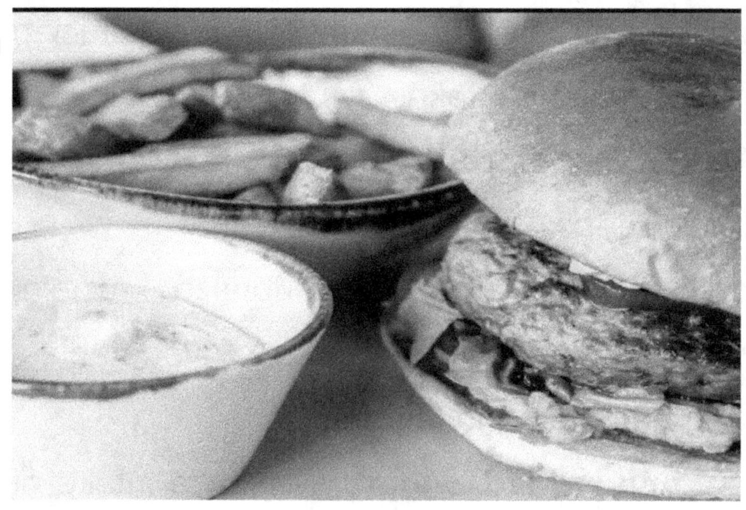

Nutrition is a fundamental aspect of maintaining a healthy lifestyle, and understanding the role of fats and essential nutrients is crucial for overall well-being. This comprehensive guide delves into the significance of fats, the various types, and the broader spectrum of essential nutrients vital for optimal bodily functions.

Fats: The Basics

1. Types of Fats:

   - **Saturated Fats**: Found in animal products and some plant oils, saturated fats, when consumed in excess, may contribute to cardiovascular issues.

   - **Unsaturated Fats**:

- **Monounsaturated Fats**: Olive oil, avocados, and nuts are rich sources, promoting heart health.

- **Polyunsaturated Fats**: Essential fatty acids, including omega-3 and omega-6, play a critical role in brain function and reducing inflammation.

2. Role of Fats:

- **Energy Source**: Fats serve as a concentrated energy source, aiding in the absorption of fat-soluble vitamins (A, D, E, and K).

- **Cellular Structure**: Fats are integral components of cell membranes, influencing cell integrity and function.

- **Hormone Production**: Certain fats are precursors to hormone synthesis, contributing to hormonal balance.

3. Dietary Recommendations:

- Balancing fat intake is key; opting for healthier fats and limiting saturated and trans fats is advisable.

- Incorporating sources like fish, nuts, seeds, and plant oils provides a well-rounded fat profile.

Essential Nutrients: An Overview

1. Macronutrients:

- **Proteins**: Comprising amino acids, proteins are vital for tissue repair, immune function, and enzyme production.

- **Carbohydrates**: Mainly providing energy, complex carbohydrates from whole grains, fruits, and vegetables offer sustained fuel.

2. Micronutrients:

- **Vitamins**: Essential for various physiological processes, vitamins come in water-soluble (B, C) and fat-soluble (A, D, E, K) forms.

  - Minerals: Critical for bone health, nerve function, and enzyme activity, minerals include calcium, iron, potassium, and zinc.

3. Water:

  - Often overlooked, water is a vital nutrient, supporting digestion, nutrient transport, and temperature regulation.

 Ensuring a Balanced Diet

1. Variety is Key:

  - A diverse diet ensures a broad spectrum of nutrients, reducing the risk of deficiencies.

2. Portion Control:

  - Moderation in portion sizes helps maintain a healthy balance of nutrients, preventing excess calorie intake.

3. Individualized Needs:

- Factors such as age, sex, activity level, and health conditions influence nutrient requirements. Tailoring nutrition to individual needs is essential.

In conclusion, fats and essential nutrients play pivotal roles in sustaining life and promoting health. A balanced diet, rich in a variety of nutrient sources, is the cornerstone of a robust nutritional foundation, contributing to overall well-being and longevity.

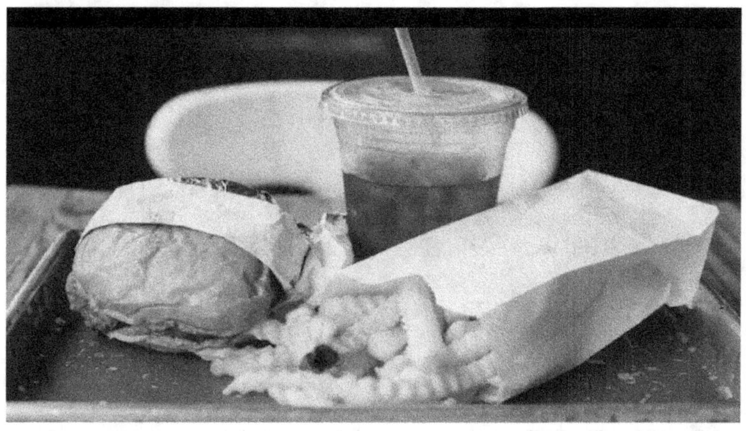

CHAPTER 4 : Incompatible Combinations

Incompatible food combinations refer to pairings of foods that may lead to digestive discomfort, nutrient absorption issues, or other health concerns. Understanding these combinations can contribute to better digestive health. Here are some examples of incompatible food combinations:

1. **Fruits with Proteins**: Consuming fruits immediately after a protein-rich meal can be challenging for digestion. Fruits typically have a quick digestion time, while proteins require a more extended period. This may

lead to fermentation in the stomach, causing bloating and discomfort.

2. Milk with Certain Foods: Milk, especially whole milk, can hinder the absorption of iron when consumed with iron-rich foods like red meat. Calcium in milk competes with iron for absorption, potentially leading to an inadequate uptake of this essential mineral.

3. Starchy Foods with Acidic Foods: Combining starchy foods (like bread or potatoes) with acidic foods (like tomatoes or citrus fruits) may cause digestive issues. The acidic environment can interfere with the enzymes responsible for starch digestion.

4. High-Protein Foods with Dairy: Pairing high-protein foods with dairy products might be challenging for some individuals. The calcium in dairy can hinder the absorption of certain proteins. It's advisable to include a variety of protein sources in the diet to ensure optimal nutrient absorption.

5. Melons with Other Foods: Melons, especially watermelon, should ideally be consumed separately from other foods. Mixing melons with other fruits or meals can lead to fermentation in the digestive tract, causing bloating and discomfort.

6. Caffeine with Calcium-Rich Foods: Excessive consumption of caffeine, found in coffee and tea, can interfere with the absorption of calcium. It's recommended to moderate caffeine intake, especially when consuming calcium-rich foods or supplements.

7. Sugary Foods with Starchy Foods: Combining sugary foods with starchy foods may lead to a rapid spike in blood sugar levels. This can strain the body's insulin response and contribute to long-term health issues like insulin resistance.

8. Different Protein Types Together: Mixing various types of protein in one meal, such as combining animal and plant-based proteins, might pose challenges for digestion. Each protein type requires specific enzymes for breakdown, and combining them can lead to inefficient digestion.

Understanding these incompatible food combinations is crucial for promoting optimal digestion and nutrient absorption. However, individual tolerance may vary, and it's always advisable to listen to your body's signals and consult with a healthcare professional or nutritionist for personalized advice.

Avoiding Conflicting Food Groups

Avoiding conflicting food groups is essential for maintaining a balanced and healthy diet. When planning meals, it's crucial to understand the principles of food compatibility to optimize nutrient absorption and promote overall well-being.

Understanding Conflicting Food Groups:

1. Protein and Starches:

- **Issue**: Consuming high-protein and high-starch foods together can lead to digestive discomfort.

- **Solution**: Separate protein and starch-rich foods to aid in better digestion.

2. Fruits and Proteins:

- **Issue**: Fruits are quickly digested, while proteins take longer, causing digestive issues when consumed together.

- **Solution**: Eat fruits on an empty stomach or as a snack between meals.

3. Milk and Certain Fruits:

- **Issue**: Some fruits can cause curdling when combined with milk, leading to digestive problems.

- **Solution**: Consume milk separately or choose fruits that don't interact negatively.

Tips for Avoiding Conflicting Food Combinations:

1. Space Out Meals:

- Allow sufficient time between meals to ensure proper digestion and nutrient absorption.

2. Understand Digestive Time:

- Different foods require varying digestion times. Pair foods with similar digestion rates to avoid conflicts.

3. Consider Food Categories:

- Categorize foods into groups (proteins, carbohydrates, fruits, etc.) and plan meals accordingly.

4. Combine Smartly:

- Pair foods that complement each other, such as vegetables with proteins or fats.

Sample Balanced Meal Ideas:

1. Grilled Chicken with Vegetables:

- Combining lean protein with non-starchy vegetables ensures a balanced and easily digestible meal.

2. Quinoa Salad with Avocado:

- A combination of a complete protein (quinoa) with healthy fats (avocado) and vegetables makes for a nutritious and harmonious dish.

Benefits of Avoiding Conflicting Food Groups:

1. Improved Digestion:

   - Minimizing conflicting food combinations reduces digestive stress and promotes better nutrient absorption.

2. Stable Blood Sugar Levels:

   - Balancing macronutrients helps regulate blood sugar levels, promoting sustained energy throughout the day.

3. Enhanced Nutrient Utilization:

   - Optimal food pairing ensures that the body efficiently utilizes the nutrients present in the diet.

Conclusion:

In conclusion, being mindful of food combinations is crucial for maintaining a harmonious and nutritious diet. By understanding the principles of food compatibility and following simple guidelines, individuals can promote better digestion, nutrient absorption, and overall health.

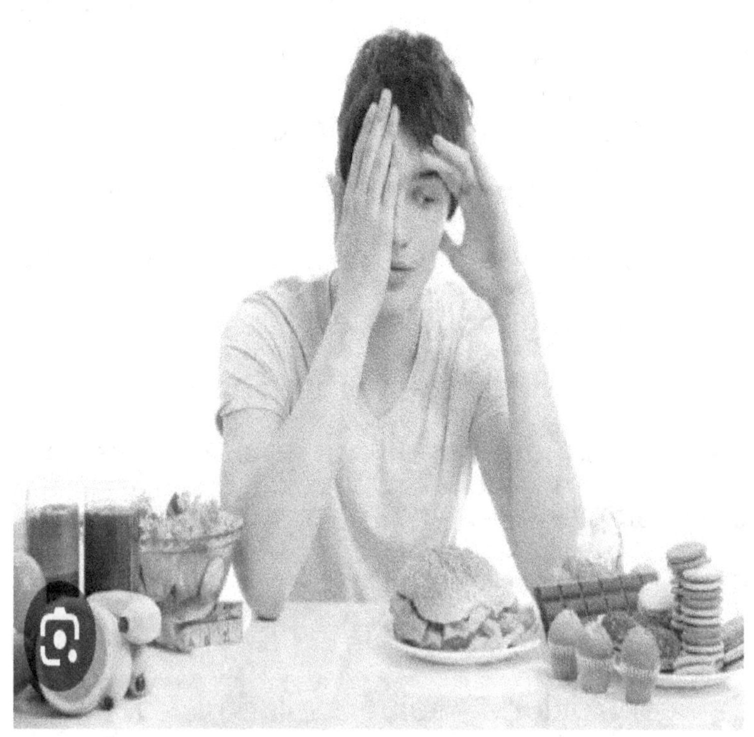

Common Mistakes in Food Combining

Food combining is a dietary practice that involves consuming certain types of foods together to optimize digestion and nutrient absorption. However, several common mistakes can compromise the effectiveness of this approach:

1. Mixing Proteins and Starches: Combining proteins (such as meat, fish, or eggs) with starches (like bread, pasta, or rice) can lead to digestive issues. Proteins require an acidic environment for digestion, while starches need an alkaline one. Mixing the two may result in inefficient digestion and discomfort.

2. Fruit After Meals: Consuming fruits immediately after a meal can hinder digestion. Fruits have a faster transit time through the digestive tract, and when eaten after heavier foods, they may ferment, leading to bloating and gas.

3. Wrong Fats with Carbohydrates: Pairing fats with carbohydrates can slow down digestion. For instance, combining a high-fat sauce with pasta can lead to prolonged digestion and potential discomfort.

4. Eating Too Quickly: Rushing through meals can hinder proper food breakdown. Chewing food thoroughly aids digestion, and skipping this step may lead to undigested food particles entering the stomach.

5. Dairy with Acidic Fruits: Mixing dairy and acidic fruits (such as oranges or tomatoes) can disrupt digestion. The acid in fruits can curdle the proteins in dairy, causing digestive discomfort.

6. Multiple Protein Sources in One Meal: Combining various protein sources in a single meal, like eating both meat and dairy, can overwhelm the digestive system. Each protein type requires specific enzymes for digestion.

7. Incompatible Food Temperatures: Consuming foods at extreme temperatures, like cold and hot items together, can disturb digestion. It's advisable to aim for foods at a moderate temperature to support the body's digestive processes.

8. Overeating: Regardless of food combining principles, excessive food intake can strain the digestive system. It's crucial to listen to your body's hunger and fullness cues to avoid overeating.

9. Ignoring Individual Tolerances: Food combining guidelines are not one-size-fits-all. Individual tolerance varies, and certain combinations that work for some may not be suitable for others. Pay attention to your body's responses to different food combinations.

10. Drinking During Meals: Consuming large amounts of liquid during meals can dilute stomach acid, potentially impacting digestion. It's advisable to drink water between meals rather than with them.

In conclusion, while food combining can be beneficial for some, it's essential to be mindful of individual differences and preferences. Experimenting with various combinations and paying attention to your body's responses can help determine what works best for you.

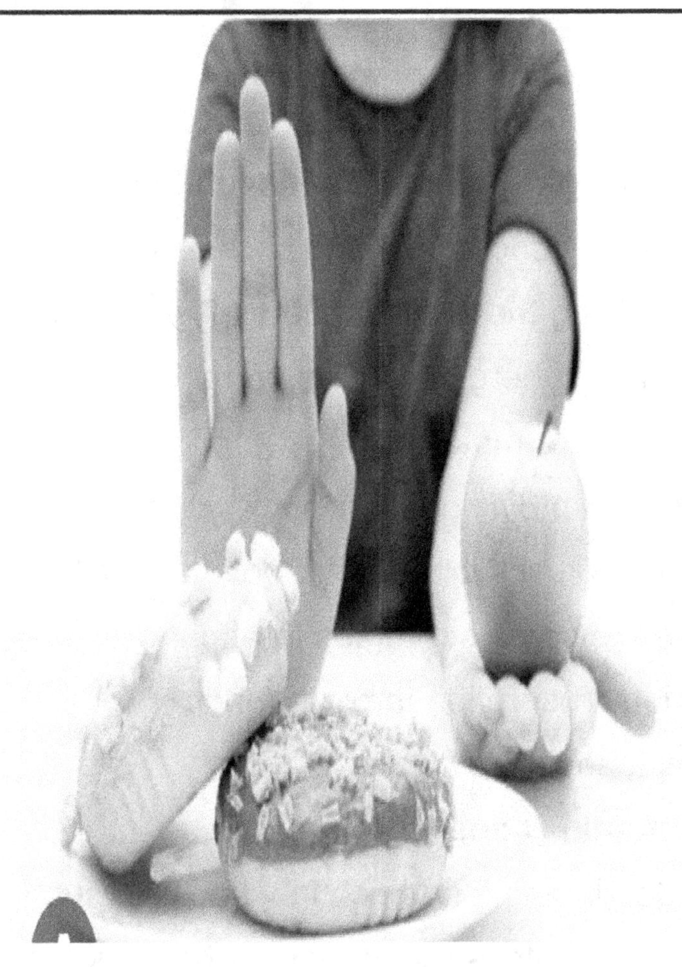

CHAPTER 5: Enhancing Nutrient Absorption

Enhancing nutrient absorption through thoughtful food combinations is essential for maximizing the nutritional benefits of your diet. The synergy between certain foods can significantly improve the absorption of key nutrients, providing your body with the building blocks it needs for optimal health. Here are some strategies to enhance nutrient absorption through food combinations:

1. Vitamin C and Iron:

   - Combining foods rich in vitamin C, such as citrus fruits, strawberries, or bell peppers, with iron-rich foods like spinach or lean meats enhances the absorption of nonheme iron. This is particularly beneficial for individuals following a plant-based diet.

2. Healthy Fats and Fat-Soluble Vitamins:

   - Pairing foods containing healthy fats (avocado, olive oil, nuts) with sources of fat-soluble vitamins (vitamin A, D, E, and K found in vegetables, dairy, and fish) aids in the absorption of these vitamins. This is because fat-soluble vitamins require fat for optimal absorption.

3. Turmeric and Black Pepper:

   - Curcumin, the active compound in turmeric, has enhanced absorption when combined with black pepper, which contains piperine. This combination increases the bioavailability of curcumin, known for its

anti-inflammatory and antioxidant
properties.

4. Calcium and Vitamin D:

- Calcium absorption is improved when combined with vitamin D. Foods like dairy products, fortified plant-based milks, and fatty fish are good sources of both calcium and vitamin D. This pairing supports bone health and overall immunity.

5. Protein and Vitamin B12:

- Consuming foods high in vitamin B12, such as meat, fish, or fortified cereals, with protein-rich sources enhances the absorption of this essential vitamin. This is particularly relevant for individuals with a vegetarian or vegan diet.

6. Fiber and Probiotics:

- The combination of fiber-rich foods (whole grains, fruits, vegetables) with probiotics (found in yogurt, kefir, and fermented foods) promotes gut health. Fiber provides a prebiotic environment for probiotics to thrive, aiding in better nutrient absorption and overall digestive well-being.

7. Phytate Reduction:

   - Soaking, fermenting, or sprouting grains, nuts, and seeds can reduce the phytate content. Phytates can hinder the absorption of minerals like zinc, iron, and calcium. By minimizing phytates, the bioavailability of these minerals is improved.

8. Sequential Eating:

   - Consuming raw vegetables before cooked ones in a meal can optimize enzyme availability, aiding in the breakdown and absorption of nutrients. This sequential approach supports better digestion and absorption of essential vitamins and minerals.

9. Balanced Macronutrient Intake:

   - Ensuring a balanced intake of carbohydrates, proteins, and fats in a meal helps regulate blood sugar levels, supporting the proper absorption of nutrients. This balance promotes sustained energy and overall metabolic health. Incorporating these strategies into your dietary habits can contribute to enhanced nutrient absorption, ensuring that your body efficiently utilizes the diverse range of nutrients from the foods you consume. Always consult with a healthcare professional or a registered dietitian for personalized advice based on your specific health needs and goals.

Synergistic Food Pairings

Synergistic food pairings involve combining different foods to enhance flavor, nutrition, and overall dining experience. This culinary concept extends beyond simple taste compatibility, aiming to create a harmonious blend that offers nutritional benefits and maximizes the bioavailability of nutrients.

1. Flavor Harmony:

- Synergistic pairings often focus on complementing and contrasting flavors. For example, the sweetness of honey with the savory notes of cheese or the acidity of tomatoes with the richness of olive oil creates a balanced and enjoyable taste experience.

2. Nutrient Optimization:

   - Combining foods strategically can enhance the absorption of nutrients. For instance, pairing spinach with vitamin C-rich fruits, like strawberries or citrus, can increase the absorption of iron from spinach due to the vitamin C content.

3. Protein Complementation:

   - Vegetarians and vegans often use synergistic food pairings to ensure they obtain complete proteins. Combining legumes with grains, such as beans and rice, provides a complementary amino acid profile, resulting in a more balanced and nutritious meal.

4. Bioavailability Boost:

- Certain nutrients are better absorbed when consumed together. For instance, pairing foods rich in fat-soluble vitamins (like vitamin A, D, E, and K) with healthy fats, such as avocados or nuts, can enhance the absorption of these vitamins.

5. Culinary Creativity:

- Synergistic pairings encourage culinary experimentation and creativity. Chefs often explore unique combinations, like balsamic vinegar with strawberries or chocolate with chili, to surprise and delight the palate.

6. Balanced Meals:

- Crafting meals with a variety of food groups ensures a balanced nutritional intake. Pairing complex carbohydrates with lean proteins, healthy fats, and a colorful array of vegetables contributes to a well-rounded and satisfying meal.

7. Cultural Significance:

   - Many traditional cuisines have evolved to incorporate synergistic food pairings based on cultural practices and regional ingredients. These pairings often have historical significance and contribute to the identity of a particular culinary tradition.

8. Mindful Eating:

   - Synergistic pairings can promote mindful eating by encouraging individuals to savor and appreciate the combination of flavors. This approach fosters a deeper connection with food and may contribute to better digestion and overall satisfaction.

9. Health Benefits:

   - Some synergistic pairings are known for their specific health benefits. For example, combining turmeric with black pepper enhances the absorption of curcumin, the active compound in turmeric, known for its anti-inflammatory properties.

In summary, synergistic food pairings go beyond taste, incorporating nutritional science, cultural influences, and creative exploration. Whether for optimizing nutrient absorption, creating culinary masterpieces, or promoting overall well-being, the art of combining foods synergistically adds depth and enjoyment to the dining experience.

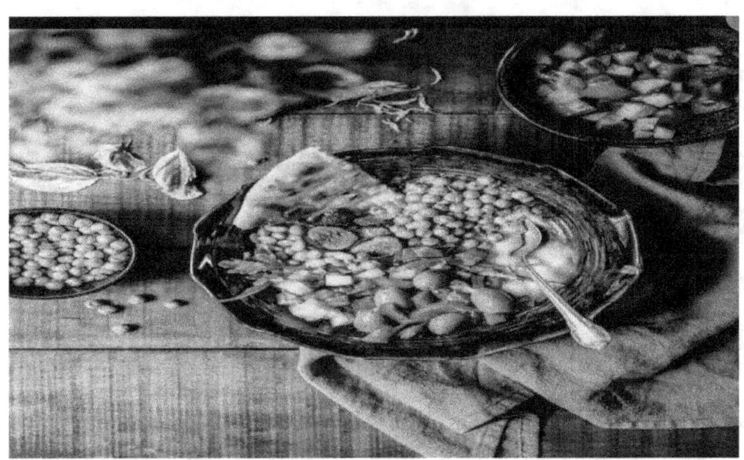

Bioavailability and Nutrient Utilization: Unveiling the Intricacies of Nutrient Absorption

Nutrient intake is a pivotal aspect of maintaining optimal health, but it's not just about what we consume; it's also about how effectively our bodies absorb and utilize these essential compounds. This intricate process is encapsulated by the concepts of bioavailability and nutrient utilization.

Understanding Bioavailability:

1. Definition:

Bioavailability refers to the proportion of a nutrient that enters the bloodstream when introduced into the body and is made available for utilization or storage. It encompasses factors influencing absorption, distribution, metabolism, and excretion of nutrients.

2. Factors Influencing Bioavailability:

- **Chemical Form**: Nutrients exist in various forms, and their chemical structure can impact absorption. For instance, iron from animal sources (heme iron) is more bioavailable than non-heme iron from plants.

-**Nutrient Interactions**: Some nutrients enhance or inhibit the absorption of others. For instance, vitamin C enhances the absorption of nonheme iron.

- **Digestive Enzymes**: Enzymes facilitate the breakdown of complex nutrients into absorbable forms. Insufficient enzyme activity can hinder bioavailability.

3. Measurement:

Bioavailability can be assessed through methods such as blood tests, urine tests, or monitoring physiological responses to nutrient intake.

Nutrient Utilization:

1. Cellular Uptake:

Once absorbed, nutrients traverse various biological barriers to reach cells. Cellular uptake involves nutrient transporters, specific proteins facilitating the entry of nutrients into cells.

2. Storage and Metabolism:

Nutrients can be stored for future use or undergo metabolic processes to generate energy. The liver plays a crucial role in metabolizing and distributing nutrients to different tissues.

3. Factors Affecting Utilization:

- **Genetic Variations**: Individual genetic makeup can influence how efficiently nutrients are utilized.

- **Health Status**: Illnesses, medications, or chronic conditions can impact nutrient utilization.

- **Age and Life Stage**: Nutrient needs and utilization vary across life stages, from infancy to old age.

Enhancing Bioavailability and Nutrient Utilization:

1. Balanced Diet:

Consuming a diverse and balanced diet ensures an adequate intake of various nutrients, optimizing bioavailability.

2. Cooking Methods:

Certain cooking methods can enhance or diminish the bioavailability of nutrients. For example, cooking tomatoes increases the absorption of lycopene.

3. Nutrient Synergy:

Pairing foods strategically can enhance nutrient absorption. For instance, combining sources of vitamin D with calcium-rich foods improves calcium utilization.

Challenges and Considerations:

1. Absorption Challenges:

Some individuals may face challenges in nutrient absorption due to digestive disorders, surgeries, or medication interactions.

2. Overnutrition and Toxicity:

Excessive intake of certain nutrients can lead to toxicity, emphasizing the importance of balance in nutrient consumption.

Conclusion:

In the intricate dance of bioavailability and nutrient utilization, understanding the science behind absorption and utilization is crucial for maintaining optimal health. By considering factors influencing bioavailability, adopting healthy eating practices, and addressing individual variations, we can unlock the full potential of the nutrients we consume, promoting overall well-being.

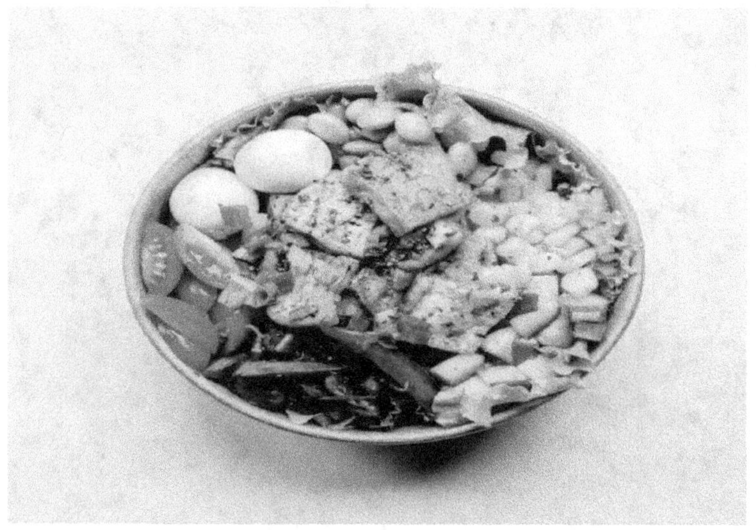

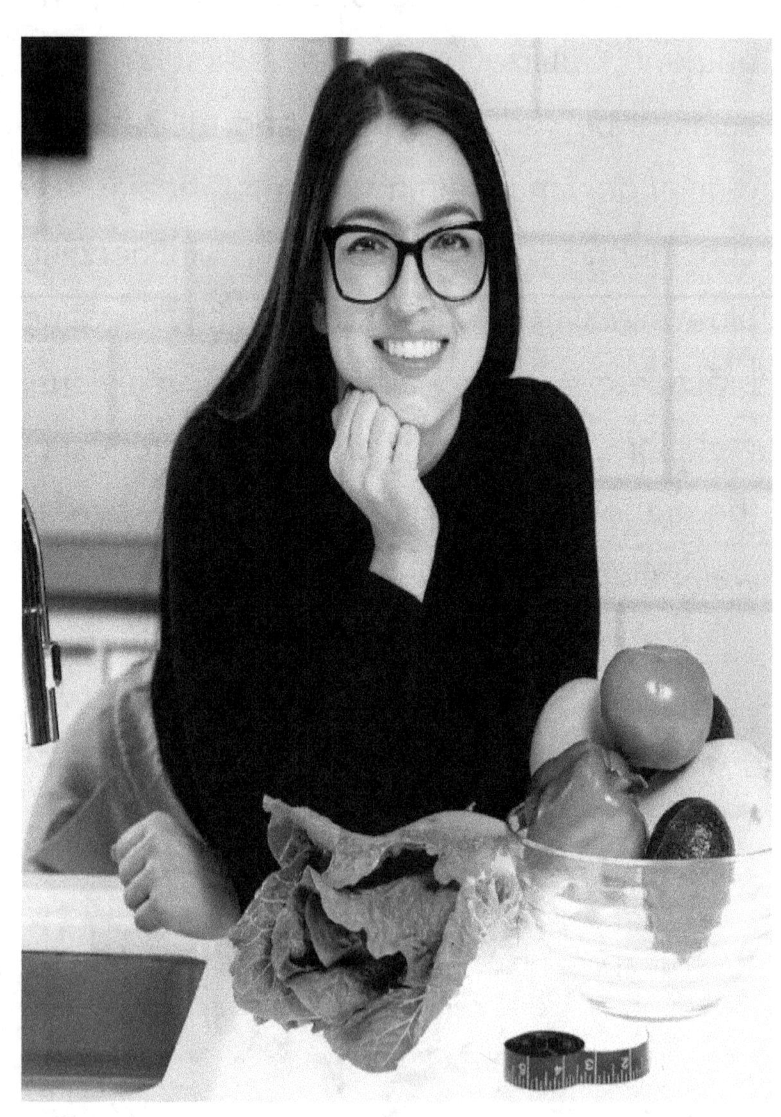

www.ingramcontent.com/pod-product-compliance
Lightning Source LLC
Chambersburg PA
CBHW070754250726
48662CB00004B/1796